A GUIDE TO 21st CENTURY ILLNESSES

Published by Rita Ferraro
Book Design by Don Shapiro
Cover Design by Steve Fata

Copyright © 2017 Rita Ferraro
All Rights Reserved
No Part of this book may be copied or reproduced in any form without the permission of the author or publisher.

ISBN: 978-1974470211

Printed in the United States of America

Disclaimer

The information contained in this book represents the personal experience and opinions of its author. The purpose of this publication is to educate the reader. All doses of supplements listed are based on the author's personal experience. It is sold and/or distributed with the understanding that the author and publisher are not responsible for any consequences, direct, or indirect, resulting from any reader's action(s).

While the author has made every effort to provide accurate sources of supplements, supplies, and internet addresses at the time of publication, neither the author nor publisher assumes the responsibility for errors or for changes that occur after this publication. This book is not intended to be a substitute for consultation with a healthcare provider.

DEDICATION

To the most compassionate man I know
whose undying love
makes life so sweet.
To my husband, Don Shapiro.

You were born with potential.
You were born with goodness and trust.
You were born with ideals and dreams.
You were born with greatness.
You were born with wings.
You are not meant for crawling, so don't.
You have wings.
Learn to use them and fly.

Rumi

TABLE OF CONTENTS

FORWARD	4
ACKNOWLEDGEMENTS	8
ABOUT THE AUTHOR	12
MY STORY	16
WELCOME TO DETOX CITY	26
HOW TO USE THIS GUIDE	27
CHAPTER 1. NUTRITION	34
CHAPTER 2 INTESTINAL SUPPORT	42
CHAPTER 3. LIVER SUPPORT	48
CHAPTER 4. EMF	67
CHAPTER 5. THE SAUNA PROGRAM	72
CHAPTER 6. PEARLS	83
CHAPTER 7. ORAL SUPPLEMENTS	92
CHAPTER 8. RECTAL USE OF SUPPLEMENTS	98
WHAT CAN I EXPECT DURING THE DETOXIFICATION PROCESS	104
WHERE DO I FIND THE SUPPLEMENTS IN THIS GUIDE	110
EPILOGUE	116
REFERENCES	119
NOTES/JOURNAL	123

FORWARD

As citizens of the country with the most wealth ever accumulated in one Nation we experience many benefits to be sure. But the best healthcare in the world is not one of those things. In fact, the United States is statistically far behind every developed country and even third world countries when it comes to quality of care compared to the massive expense per capita for health care in this country. Essentially, healthcare in this country has for some time been hijacked by pharmaceutical and other corporations, and preventing suffering and death got lost in the predatory capitalism that so often controls the laws and regulatory agencies that create American healthcare. Take a minute to think about that, the American healthcare system is behind countries like Cuba and the Czech Republic. This is not just an interesting statistic, real people and real suffering is often the outcome. People are being failed by this system.

I first met Rita Ferraro in the summer of 1996 at a clinic in Dallas, Texas. We were both fighting life threatening illnesses and soon struck up a friendship. Sometimes kindred spirits are drawn together like magnets and especially in times of crisis. Rita and I had amazingly similar medical histories and stories. Both of us sought the best medical treatment available, and were failed by the system. Both of us were told by allopathic doctors that our illness was "all in our heads", and that we were in good health, even as we were in severe pain and wasted away to nothing with emaciation. And finally, both of us suffered severe insomnia, meaning weeks on end with no sleep. We had nearly identical experiences when admitted to hospitals under suicide watch due to said insomnia, namely, once we were finally medicated enough to sleep a few hours the nurses and hospital workers continued to wake us up constantly throughout the night to ask us if we wanted to hurt ourselves or to take our vitals. Just another example of common sense being displaced by ridiculous adherence to procedure.

But to me it was not just a friend I had made, Rita quickly became a mentor in how to successfully fight for one's health after being failed by allopathic medicine, and this did not mean only "finding the right doctor". It meant gaining empowerment to fight for one's own health by taking in knowledge. In the clinic in which we met there were many patients that were sad, angry, frightened and basically just bemoaning the misfortune of illness. Rita was not this way. She was on a mission to get well and unlike myself coming from a State (Arkansas -that was a no-man's land for natural and alternative medicine at the time), she was from Manhattan and as a Psychotherapist with a background in biochemistry and a keen intelligence and ability to put complex knowledge into practical actions. Rita was sicker than most of the other patients, and also putting forth heroic effort to beat the odds.

In short, I needed her and she generously gave her time and helped me begin learning new concepts about holistic healing. I was extremely ill. Having lost from 155 lbs. down to 98 lbs. with severe mercury poisoning,

Lyme disease, and multiple intestinal parasite infections, there was no room for mistakes. In fact, Rita said those exact words. "No more mistakes Jack." I had to decide in favor of two fundamental principles at that time. Nutrition and detoxification were the only way I was going to survive. Taking toxic meds to kill infection was in fact killing me. I did not recognize this. Rita did.

I owe my life to Rita Ferraro. Without her timely and wise advice I would have almost certainly died back there in the 90's before my 30th birthday. We both liquidated real estate in excess of 100's of 1000s of dollars to fight illness outside the mainstream of medical treatment, but in many ways her common sense practical advice was more valuable than the medical help I paid for. Now I have my health back, have a degree in natural health, and have a successful traditional naturopathic practice. In a way all the people who have in turn reported benefits from my care in some way owe that to Rita. I am just paying it forward. And if Rita's knowledge could make the difference in my survival those years ago, then her current knowledge of course surpasses that considerably.

For those with the type of illnesses such as the ones we battled "SAVE YOUR LIFE" can do just that. It is sound, well researched information that empowers you to begin making rapid recovery mostly by taking your health into your own hands. It is a well-designed, and well laid out book that even the sickest, most brain fogged Chronic Fatigue, Lyme patient, or other chronically ill patient can put into practical application. It is based on the same two common sense principles that saved my life years ago: one, when your body is sick, put as many nutrients and good things in as possible, and two, eliminate as many toxins and stressors as you can simultaneously. I encourage any person who is dealing with a chronic illness that has been failed by the allopathic medical establishment to read this book, or anyone with a suffering family member to buy this book and put the methods into action right away.

Jack Miller CTN
Traditional Naturopath and owner of Natural Health Sciences of Arizona, LLC
Professor of ACIM (Academy of Comprehensive and Integrative Medicine)

ACKNOWLEDGEMENTS

Thank you Dr. Sherry Rogers for your appearance on the Carol Martin Show many moons ago. Dr. Rea, you introduced me to the detoxification of the human body. But most importantly, you believed every crazy symptom I had and validated me in a way no one else had. Christopher Rea, Dr. Rea's son, you drove my car from Texas to Santa Fe making sure that the home I rented was chemically safe for me. I am forever in your debt. You stood on my side when rough times occurred in Dallas.

A special thank you to Stephen Levine from Allergy Research/Nutricology. You made a unique product called Co-Rectalvite, with my instructions and helped people who were chronically ill receive nutrients in a less expense way than having an IV infusion. I am so privileged to call you my friend.

Jack Miller (CTN) my best friend, buddy, and grasshopper. I am so proud to be your mentor even though it is sometimes the other way around. You and I have been through thick and thin, and through hell and back. We have a bond I share with no one else. Thank you for being in my life. Thank you for introducing Laser Energetic Detoxification to me. Although it was late in my recovery, people with chronic illness can go to your amazing website and learn all about it and begin treatment early in their recovery. You are a blessing.

Carol Grohs and "the Franz" (Mr. Tweety), thank you so much for bringing joy and companionship at a time of great isolation. Your friendship is dear to me.

Regina, my twin sister, you have always been there for me from the start. Calling me on the telephone while I was in a psychiatric ward. Bewildered like me when no doctor knew what was wrong with me. You bore the pain and suffering along with me. I know how helpless you felt. Thank you for visiting me in Dallas, Santa Fe.... you, the only person I wasn't allergic to. You took time away from your own family to make sure you saw me in person. I am forever grateful.

Thank you to my family for always believing in me. You never doubted my diagnosis. My family embraces a new lifestyle, they eat organic food, and are educated in the toxicity in the world. I am proud of you Mom and Dad. Thank you to my four sisters who support me in all different ways; although we don't live close we are close.

Thank You Carolyn Parrs and Devi Records from Women as Game Changers. Enrolling in your six month training program prompted me to write this book. You helped me to believe in myself as a working woman and entrepreneur. I understand my inner and outer game because of you. I have made lifetime friends in our group. Consuelo Luz, you are one of them. You were one of two of my accountability partners. Your musical artistry touches me and so many others. I have to shout out to the talented Karen Marie Jones Meadows who was my other accountability partner. Karen you have taught me to be intimidated by no one. Your one women show on Harriet Tubman inspires me to be the best I can be. Thank you for your friendship.

Michael Payne, thank you for the great consultations we have. You are my go to man. Your passion in creating Living Well Today is exemplified by the number of patients you help and cure. You use cutting edge energy medicine that can be done remotely and set it up in a genius way. People are blessed to have you as their doctor. Your new IV clinic for NADH and nasal NADH is helping so many people as well as your customized homeopathics.

Thank you to my husband Don Shapiro who is my everything. You support me and encourage me every day, even when your life gets crazy! You will drop everything to take the cat to the Vet, rush home when my car breaks down, etc.

Yet, you still find the energy for spiritual studies, to tend our garden, play Flamenco, and stay connected to the community as a mentor and advocate for young people, and an activist for environmental justice.

ABOUT THE AUTHOR

It is 1997, I am 79 lbs. I am allergic to my bed, a pencil, a cup, people, pets, and everything known to man. I sleep in a small room on a tiled floor with a piece of barrier cloth as my bed. I am an environmental refugee. I can no longer go home to New York City. I am forced to live in the mountains of Santa Fe, New Mexico. I awake in the morning without my husband (and I actually like him) and pets. I wear an old raggedy linen shirt and pants that I have to wash every day. I am even allergic to organic cotton. I am a universal reactor.

I have lost my house twice. The first time causing me to live in the Santa Fe National Forest. The second time, I had to live on my husband's porch which was a log cabin in Edgewood, New Mexico. Uh Oh! Winter was coming, so I slept outside on my porch in a covered cloth sauna,

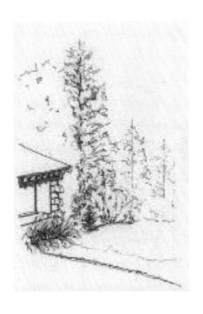

Why consider this program?
Because it saved my life, and can save yours too!
I have twenty years of experience
and success.
I am a passionate solution finder.
Eighteen years later I am a Naturopath.

➤ My book, "SAVE YOUR LIFE: A GUIDE TO DETOXIFICATION FOR 21ST CENTURY ILLNESSES is a guide to your personal recovery.

The word "guide" is used to mean that one size does not fit all. You will find you can do certain treatments in this book while other treatments do not appeal to you or your body rejects them. You may take certain parts of this book and work with those treatment strategies. The purpose of my book is to arm you with information in navigating a horrible if not impossible illness so my story does not have to be yours. It is for someone who wants to detoxify in a way that is well thought out and safe and for someone who has a hole in their program that needs to be filled in. It is for someone who is caught like a deer in the highlights hearing their illness is now chronic and there is no recovery. Here! Take these pills and eventually die.

What is purposely missing from my book is the treatment of heavy metal poisoning with chelating agents such as DMSA, DMPS and ALA. This is done on purpose. I want the body to be strong and supported by the therapies in this book before removing mercury fillings. You can have the mercury fillings removed and the necessary treatment chelation protocol afterwards.

The 2nd edition of this book will be on heavy metal toxicity and other advanced treatments. The proper techniques to remove amalgam fillings and safe ways of chelation therapy. I lost six years of my life from improper chelation of mercury. We were the pioneers that experimented on each other so that you can have a better time at it.

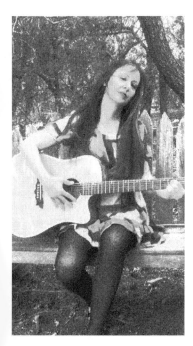

Presently, I weigh 118 lbs. I am healthy and have a life. Against all odds you can carve a life out for yourself. With willingness and hard work, you too can be healthy again. I have some chemical sensitivities, but can recover in 30 minutes. In the past it might have taken me six months.

MY STORY

I was a successful 40 year-old psychoanalytic psychotherapist practicing on New York's Fifth Avenue in Greenwich Village. I have a Master's degree in Social Work, (MSW) from New York University School of Social Work.

I began to have allergies and sinusitis. I lived on the antihistamine seldane. I visited an acupuncturist for sinus pain and was given Chinese herbs which helped but I had to go twice a week. I was diagnosed with Interstitial Cystitis and had water hydrodystention with cystoscopy performed on me in a hospital. The diagnosis was confirmed.

I purchased new bedroom furniture and carpeting and began to have insomnia and anxiety at night. My psychotherapy office was flooded from a leak in an upstairs doctor's office and we had mold growing along with contaminated fluids on the walls. I also had a microscopic cutting edge procedure on a failed root canal. Six new amalgams were also placed that year.

In my teen years, I was trained as a dental assistant as a part-time job. In my senior year, I graduated six months earlier and my job became full-time.

In those days, dental assistants made the amalgams by combining liquid mercury (that's right!) dispensed into a steel capsule with other metal powders which were placed in a machine that agitated the formula. It was then placed on a cheesecloth and presented to the dentist for approval.

If the amalgam mixture was too wet, you just squeezed the cheese cloth and excess mercury would show and be thrown on the rug. No big deal. No one told me it was poison.

I wore no gloves or protection. My brain was still developing. I had twenty one fillings at the time. The dentist felt bad that they were old and disintegrating so he took the old ones out and replaced them with shiny new amalgams.

Years later, my mom told me that when I was a child, we had been drinking contaminated well water which they wouldn't give to horses at the racetrack. She fought to put us on City water and won.

In 1997, I started having anxiety during the day and sleepless nights. I carried on with my practice as long as I could. During the session with the last patient I ever saw, I excused myself to vomit and crapped my brains out and then returned to listening. When I arrived home, I collapsed on the living room floor.

> The "Big Bang" happened...

I entered a depression that was likened by a New York Hospital psychiatrist to that of Virginia Wolfe.

I had been treated for depression and anxiety by a New York psychiatrist who was very well-known. He was even on the cover of a New Yorker Magazine with another psychiatrist. To make a long story short, he had limited experience in medication management …psychopharmacology.

Every time he prescribed an antidepressant, he would take me off the medication because of minor side-effects which could have easily been corrected.

He prescribed so many tranquilizers and barbiturates, for sleep, that the depression worsened. When I took the barbiturates my brain felt as if fireworks were exploding in it. It was horrifying! I went to see two other psychiatrists who couldn't help me.

He then prescribed lithium and I became lithium poisoned. I was misdiagnosed. No one knew I had Multiple Chemical Sensitivity with mercury poisoning. I finally came upon a psychiatrist – a skilled psycho-pharmacologist, who was affiliated with Columbia Presbyterian Hospital. Ironically, his office was across the hallway from the doctor who was poisoning me. In fact, they were colleagues.

Once he saw me he couldn't believe my history with psychiatrists and was appalled by my previous psychiatrist's treatment strategy.

When he gave me a gentle push I fell into the wall. He told my husband, Don, that I had the equivalent of a case of beer in my head from all the medications I was taking. He recommended that I be hospitalized immediately for detoxification of medications to find the right antidepressant. I had a choice of Columbia Presbyterian in Harlem or Payne Whitney Hospital in Midtown Manhattan.

I chose Payne Whitney so that Don could visit without travelling so far. I had a tendency to make it easier for others than for myself, something I never do now. I come first.

So, I lost my Columbia Presbyterian doctor. I spent 30 days in the Payne Whitney psychiatric ward. It was one of the worst experiences of my life. I was detoxed from my medications in a cruel manner. I quickly learned that no one could help me. No one! Not the best intentioned doctors. Not the best that money could buy at the time. Not my husband, parents or sisters. I was alone. I was misdiagnosed.

> **As I lay in my hospital bed, I thought,
> "God, is this the way I'm going out in my life?"**

I was discharged after a one month stay. As I lay at home, convalescing in my bed, I turned on a TV program called "Alive and Wellness," with Carol Martin. A most extraordinary female physician was featured. Her name was Sherry Rogers, M.D. She talked of a cure for

Crohn's Disease. I wanted to buy her book, *"Wellness Against All Odds."* I just had to purchase that book and find out where she practiced. Maybe she could cure Interstitial Cystitis!

There was no mention that she was a physician practicing Environmental Medicine, who herself had Multiple Chemical Sensitivity (MCS.) While anxiously waiting for her phone number to be provided at the end of the program, suddenly, cable reception went out in lower Manhattan. How could this be? What a cruel joke! No internet in those days, and it took me three days to find the book and locate where she practiced. The rest is history! I read her book feverishly.

"Oh My God?" I have "Environmental Illness."

Don arrived home from work to find our new (toxic formaldehyde - based) bedroom furniture piled up in the hallway and I lived on the twenty seventh floor of a skyscraper. He couldn't believe it but was very patient with me. I was so excited to tell him I was environmentally ill. I asked him to read Dr. Roger's book and he did. He supported me from that day forward.

I made an appointment to visit her in Syracuse, NY. I was so, so thin and sick. I collapsed in the airport, only to have three men lift me up off the floor.

Dr. Roger's recommendation was that I had to make plans to go to the *Environmental Health Center* in Dallas, Texas under the care of Dr. William Rea, M.D.

His diagnosis was Mercury Poisoning with Toxic Encephalopathy causing chemical sensitivity and chronic fatigue.

Basically, I had a brain injury. I was treated at the Center every day for 6 months. I learned so much. I began with sauna treatments, and I.V. Vitamin infusions. My immune system was that of an AIDS patient. Originally, I was to have a feeding tube inserted, but Dr. Rea said, "Let's wait two weeks and see if the treatments take effect."

I picked up so quickly, I believe, because the sauna detoxified the many medications I had been poisoned by. Dr. Rea was delighted! One day I noticed white powder on my shin. I stupidly licked it. Holy Crap!

It was fixer solution, I used when I was a dental assistant to process X- rays. I showed Dr. Rea and he casually said, "That's what happens. It's normal." I quickly washed it off.

There were no cell phones, laptops, iPads, Kindles, Wi-Fi etc., back then. Thank goodness! While at Dr. Rea's clinic, I rented an apartment at the Dallas Marriott Residence Inn where there was a microwave oven. I never owned one in New York because I read a negative article and had believed it. I experimented with the microwave and turned it on and began to feel waves of energy crashing at my body. I say waves because it felt like I was in an ocean of energy that I could not see but only feel. *Holy cow! It was so weird.* I tried to hide in a corner of the room far away from the microwave but the waves found me. I ran to the microwave and shut it off. What a crazy experience. I was so fragile and so sensitive.

Carolyn Gorman, the counselor at the Center recommended that I not return to New York. She said the state with the best rate of recovery for MCS was New Mexico. So, Don picked me up in Dallas and took me on a plane to Santa Fe, New Mexico where he had rented a house in the mountains. We really didn't appreciate the gravity of how ill I was back then.

My new home had been previously occupied by an environmentally ill woman. Nevertheless, before flying to Santa Fe, Dr. Rea's son Chris Rea, drove my car from Dallas to Santa Fe and met my husband to make sure that the house was safe. I owe a lot to Chris. My husband removed carpeting from the bedroom and had it tiled.

He made arrangements with a Wild Oats natural foods grocery store to deliver food regularly as I was too chemically sensitive to go out. Don had to immediately fly back to New York to work. I was alone on some mountain in Santa Fe, New Mexico.

As I lay on the tiled floor in my room, three phrases repeatedly came to mind. Some Jungians would call it the "Collective Unconscious." They were: "There is always a solution," "Where's there's a will, there's a way," and "God helps those who help themselves."

Another thing happened to me. The song Amazing Grace played over and over in my head twenty four seven. At first it was nice but eventually I was angry at Grace. LOL. My husband wasn't able to live with me because I had an allergy to human dander and sounds startled me.

Along with being chemically sensitive I was electromagnetically sensitive. I couldn't stand in front of my refrigerator without vibrating, use a blow dryer, TV, computer, or any equipment that had to be plugged in. I used a retro Bakelite telephone but couldn't talk on it for more than five minutes.

One of the best days living in Santa Fe was when my husband devised a box outside my window and put the TV in there. I remember watching "The Rosie O'Donnell Show" every day at four o'clock. She was my respite.

A shout out to Rosie whose show really helped me laugh. I finally bought a cotton futon and was able to sleep on it. No more achy bones. Yay!

I continued my detox program and sang to myself every day. My pet was a spider I called "Spidey." He stayed with me in the same spot for a year.

In Santa Fe I got well enough to go outside and lay in my hammock. One day I heard the loudest buzzing.

I jumped out of the hammock as I thought a motor cycle was coming to run me over. It was just a Hummingbird. I was so embarrassed. I had never seen or heard a hummingbird before. It flew so close to me. Remember I was very sensitive to sound.

After 3 years, I moved into a house in Edgewood, New Mexico where I was reunited with my husband and three cats, but of course I slept outside on the porch. The house wasn't safe for me yet. In the morning the outside wooden door opened to a screened door – and behind it, my cats greeted me. I'd say, "Hello, good morning munchkins!" Can you believe they lived inside and I lived outside! How crazy!

Eventually with continued treatment I wormed my way inside, first to shower, then to cook and finally to sleep. I lived inside. Awesome! And no allergy to my husband and cats. What a win! My detox program had made a difference! We lived there for about a year until we found a house in Cedar Crest, New Mexico where I continue to thrive and where I can forest bathe every day. We do have four seasons. I live 8,000 ft. above sea level in a forested area. We are very grateful.

Every night I go to sleep, I thank my Lucky Stars that I have a roof over my head

WELCOME TO DETOX CITY... YOUR RECOVERY BOOTCAMP!

A DAY IN DETOX CITY

Theron Randolph, MD., the great pioneer of Clinical Ecology believed that illness is caused when the body's ability to detoxify environmental stressors is overloaded. Single, intermittent exposure to chemicals may cause no obvious harm, but if the exposure is repeated, the immune system can be overwhelmed, even at low levels.

For example, painters occupationally exposed to volatile organic compounds (VOC's) were found to have significantly more adverse reactions to VOC's than non-painters, even though the individual exposures were below the accepted threshold for harmful effects.

Dr. Randolph's concept is known as the "total load theory," or the more popular 'rain barrel effect.'

It is when more toxins enter the barrel than the body can detoxify and excrete, the barrel overflows and symptoms develop.

This explains why some people may react to environmental toxins while others do not.

HOW TO USE THIS GUIDE

I've designed this GUIDE to make it user friendly somewhat like a cookbook. It is divided into 8 chapters, with each chapter covering a key step to recovery. At the end of the book, you will find references, products and supplements described in the chapters and an idea of where to purchase them, and a few "Notes/Journal" pages to keep a record of your progress, or jot down important reminders.

Chapter 7, "Oral Supplements" provides a list, including directions for their ideal use. I do not profit from any brand supplements or products. Product brands are specifically recommended because they meet the following criteria:

- ✓ I use them and found them to be safe and effective.
- ✓ They meet the special requirements of most chemically sensitive people; purity and less fillers.
- ✓ They are reasonably priced.
- ✓ Accessibility: You can find most of them at health food stores or on the internet.

Before Beginning This Detox Program

For the first 7 weeks, make detoxification a priority. Put your stake in the ground. If you are healthier and work, take one to three weeks off and do this program.

It's your health we are talking about and prevention is the best medicine.

During the detoxification program avoid all chemicals, as well as any foods you are allergic to as much as you can.

AVOIDANCE! AVOIDANCE! & MORE AVOIDANCE! STAY HOME!

Before beginning any detoxification program, it is important to know a little bit of the methylation cycle. You need to know whether you are a CBS Upregulator because, if you are then certain steps have to be followed before a detoxification program can be implemented. CBS Upregulator is abbreviated by CBS++ or CBS+-- C699T C1080T, called Cystathionine Beta Synthase which are key enzymes of the Methylation Cycle.

It is beyond the scope of his book to talk about other mutations in the methylation cycle. If you are CBS++ or CBS+- the necessary nutrients to run the methylation cycle just go down the drain. It's like the flood gates are open. You will get sick when supplementing with certain detoxifying nutrients I recommend in this book. It's a waste of money and time. If you want more information on the methylation cycle purchase "The Puzzle of Autism" and "Genetic Bypass" by Amy Yasko, ND. Research has shown that "brain fog" is often seen in the chemically sensitive who carry the CBS++ or CBS+- mutations. I am attempting to simplify a much complex system.

HOW DO I KNOW IF I AM A CBS UPREGULATOR?

You can buy a $99.00 test online test called 23 & Me. I've seen a special at BestBuy as low as $29.00. They say they do not interpret the test, however a sister site called Genetic Genie.org will accept your account and give you the information about your methylation cycle gene mutations. Please give a donation. They will tell you your ancestry as well. Fun! But not the point. Look at the CBS status. You can also go to Dr. Amy Yasko's website www.holisticheal.com and purchase her genetic test kit which is more expensive but it comes with an interpretation.

CBS Upregulators cannot tolerate sulfur or lipid donors. They create too much ammonia which depletes other enzymes to balance neurotransmitters. Excess ammonia is very toxic in the body. Glutathione is low. Taurine is too high. Sulfur can activate the stress/cortisone reaction, increasing adrenaline and decreasing dopamine and/or epinephrine. Cortisol reaction can change magnesium, and calcium levels, decrease serotonin and dopamine and phosphatidyl serine levels and the gaba/glutamine ratio. Increased glutamate is undesirable.

CBS Upregulators need glutathione but they are in a double bind. You can't take glutathione even though you need it! CBS Upregulators cannot handle sulfur and are usually sulfur toxic and sensitive to sulfur.

CBS C699 is a "trump card" in that it overrides any other mutations and can deplete intermediate pathways. I created a list of "What to do if I am a CBS Upregulator" because many chemically sensitive people find it impossible to interpret Amy's two books because of brain fog.

THANK YOU! DR. YASKO!

WHAT DO I DO IF I AM A CBS UPREGULATOR? FOLLOW THIS ONE MONTH PROGRAM

- ✓ Do not eat cruciferous vegetables such as broccoli, cabbage, cauliflower, kale, brussel sprouts, turnips, bokchoy, watercress, radish, kohlrabi, and rapini. Avoid garlic, arugula, coconut milk, juice and oil, horseradish, mustard greens, wine and grapes.

- ✓ Have a low protein diet, preferably chicken and turkey. Avoid dairy (except butter), eggs, legumes, and beansprouts.

- ✓ Do not supplement with taurine.

- ✓ Avoid supplements such as glutathione, alpha lipoic acid, chondroitin sulfate, Cysteine, DMPS, DMSA, DMSO, Epsom Salts (bath), garlic, glucosamine sulfate, magnesium sulfate, methionine, milk thistle, MSN, NAC, taurine, and any sulfur-containing medications (antibiotics, sulfonylurea, Bactrim, all diuretics, except spironolactone.)

- ✓ Avoid food additives such as sulfur dioxide, sodium sulfite, sodium bisulfate, sodium metasulfite, potassium bisulfite, and potassium metasulfite.

- ✓ Turmeric is not high in sulfur, but it has been found to raise sulfur levels significantly, but no one knows why.

- ✓ Use SPARGA by NutraMedix to help detox sulfur.

- ✓ Only if tolerated, you can add molybdenum, GABA, L-citrulline, grape seed extract, cherry fruit extract, yucca, l-carnitine, CoQ10 and Royal Jelly.

- ✓ Nightly use of BIND or Activated Charcoal should be taken away from food.

- ✓ You can check your level of sulfur during the month by using strips sold at Holisticheal.com or CTL Scientific strips on the internet. Do not become impatient. People have told me it took them two months to decrease sulfur levels. During the CBS++ program, they noticed increased rotten egg odors in stools. It's rather noticeable. LOL

CHAPTER 1
NUTRITION

Eat fresh organic uncontaminated food. Avoid plastic containers or using frozen food in plastic bags for now. Never drink water out of a plastic bottle, or you may be adding to your toxic load.

Dr. Herbert J. Rinkel, in 1934, devised the Rotary diversified diet for people with food sensitivities. It's based on a 4-day rotation diet whereby the individual doesn't repeat a given food in a four day period. Four days was used because it generally represented maximum bowel transit time. This means that the food antigen is gone systemically from the body and won't produce a reaction. Some environmental doctors suggest you do a longer rotation if you are very toxic. I know people who successfully used this technique and did well while others had so few foods (maybe 3 or 4) and did not.

In the beginning I could only eat two foods, beef and broccoli. I sometimes ate them every day and didn't become allergic to them. Then I introduced Partridge and acorn squash and rotated them every other day.

A clever idea was brought to me by a man who would take glutamine, quercetin, homeopathic histamine and digestive enzymes before eating anything. People have told me that it worked for them.

Dr. Peter J. D'Adamo with Catherine Whitney have a book, "Eat Right for Your Type." It is a diet based on your blood-type. I like the book and recommend that you try it. I used it for a period of time.

> Do the best you can.

Some people with MCS are allergy tested through intradermal testing. You are injected until the technician finds your endpoint and that is your antigen dose. You inject the antigens subcutaneously (specific to the allergic foods) which enables you to eat those foods.

I used this technique after I finished the sauna protocol at The Environmental Health Center in Dallas, Texas. I found it to be very hard on my body. I didn't feel very well when testing. I went home from Dallas with $2,000 worth of food antigens. One morning I injected myself before breakfast and had a bright red lump at the site and I also had a fever of 103 degrees.

What I wasn't told was that it was likely that the dead measles or other dead viruses were used to carry the antigens in the body. In a phone conversation way back when, Dr. Sherry Rogers confirmed it when I told her what happened. She said, "That and whatever other viruses." I thought the injections were pure but later found out about carrier viruses. My body recognized the virus and I became ill. It disappeared after a few days.

So, the end of antigens and back to eating fewer foods. A much safer approach is to use antigens or a neutralizing dose sublingually.

I learned from a colleague that the Environmental Health Center in Dallas is presently using sublingual drops for the sensitive patient.

There are food allergy tests you can Google on the Internet, such as the Elisa test. You can get some idea of what to stay away from and what you can rotate.

There are two treatments that can effectively reverse food allergies. They are N.A.E.T. and BioSet. N.A.E.T. was one of the first energetic techniques developed by Devi Nambutripad. Practitioners were trained by Devi.

I didn't do well with N.A.E.T perhaps because of the level of expertise or experience of my practitioner. She told me that I passed car exhaust and I hadn't. I got very sick after that treatment and quit.

I became a certified BioSet practitioner while still being sick. I dragged myself to the BioSet trainings in Dallas, Texas taught by Ellen Cutler, DC: Where there is a will, there's a way! Right! I used software (IQS) installed in my computer.

This was a better technique for me because the testing revealed whether you are able to pass the treatment, although it is very difficult to test yourself. I suggest that you find a certified BioSet practitioner.

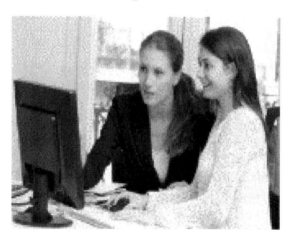

There are also Laser Sweeps using food vials to neutralize food allergies. This technique works as well. Your vial is placed in a laser device and pointed at the patient using a technique developed by Dr. Lee Cowden. It is part of a longer LED (Laser Energetic Detoxification) technique that is done with an Asyra or Zyto device.

To understand LED and Laser Sweep treatments visit NaturalHealthSciencesofArizona.com. Jack Miller Certified Traditional Naturopath walks you through a video and photos of the technique and what an LED is. It wasn't until I had LED treatments by Jack Miller that I was able to excrete mercury without very harsh side effects for the first time. I slept 3 hours during the day of that treatment, which was not possible for me back then. Any previous attempts at chelation using oral DMSA in the past just made me suicidal.

One other approach is to follow is a rare foods diet, such as the one described in "Wellness Against All Odds," by Sherry Rogers, M.D. When I introduced teff, quinoa, amaranth, goose, duck, and venison, to my diet I crashed! While it actually worked for some people, I just got sicker.

I am surprised by the number of environmentally ill people who are eating fish. Salmon has Omega 3 fish oil but it is also likely to contain mercury. You see, mercury is the 2nd most toxic element on the planet. You cannot afford to ingest even trace amounts. During my Detox program one should not eat seafood even if it is Alaskan Wild Caught Salmon.

Some people with MCS do well with butter. Another alternative is Ghee. Acceptable sweeteners are xylitol, stevia and erythritol.

> Digestive enzymes should be taken before each meal.

There are many good plant-based enzymes on the market. There are also pancreatic enzymes. Some people are deficient in hydrochloric acid in the stomach. An enzyme with betaine HCL can help with digestion. Heartburn can actually be caused by having a deficiency of stomach acid.

I am not recommending one diet over another. There are many options available. Paleo, GAPS, Vegan, Pituitary diet, and eating according to your blood type, etc. Choose the one that makes you feel best. There are energetic devices that will recommend a diet for you. Whenever I was tested, on the Zyto machine, the Pituitary Diet was selected. It meant I should eat meat including red meat. It makes sense in that mercury toxic individuals are required to eat meat while detoxing or chelating heavy metals.

I advise juicing as much as possible.

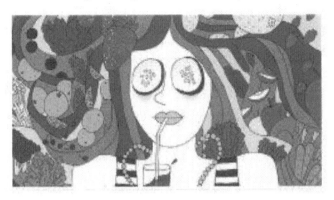

Start slow with one vegetable at a time and work up to more vegetable combinations. In no time you will begin to create delicious juices. The best juicer is one that you will use. It has to be easy for you to use and clean; otherwise, you won't use it.

Some people think you must buy a Champion juicer which is expensive and hard to clean and assemble. I know juicing gurus, who use the white/stainless steel Jack LaLane juicer for a fraction of the price. We are taught to drink the juice as soon as it is prepared, that is optimal, but you can store it in a bottled container and save it for later. Some people use a juicer twice and then sell it on Craigslist, the internet or through ads in a health food store.

Don't hesitate to buy one!
My first juicer was a used Acme.

CHAPTER 2
INTESTINAL SUPPORT

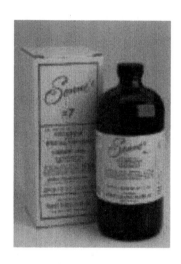

> On a colon cleanse day, eat very little. Liquids would be best for 24 hours.

I started with a very gentle colon cleanse using Bernard Jensen's technique. Today, everyone and her/his mother is selling colon cleanse kits which are very expensive and contain too many ingredients for the chemically sensitive individual. Use Sonne's #7 (Bentonite solution) and Sonne's #9 (Psyllium powder.)

In a bottle with a screw top:

- ✓ Mix 1 tablespoon Bentonite (Sonne's #7) liquid with 1 tablespoon (Sonne's #9) Psyllium powder, in 8 oz. of clean filtered water. If you cannot find Sonne's products, you may substitute another brand of Bentonite and Psyllium.

- ✓ Shake it vigorously for 15 seconds.

- ✓ Drink it all.

Since I was not able to eat many foods, I shed black sausage-like casings in the shape of intestines. I took photos of it because I couldn't believe it! This is called the mucoid layer or plaque.

LEAKY GUT

How do I know if I have it? You can take expensive tests or realize that if you are chronically ill, you probably have it!

What do I do? First, you must clean up your diet. No gluten for the time being; no dairy except butter or ghee; no sugar; no yeast products, no allergenic foods, and you must be on a rotation diet. Read every label.

L-Glutamine is the nutrient known for healing a leaky gut. There will be some people who will become too excited on the supplement. If so, discontinue.

Order a pure glutamine powder that dissolves in water and drink first thing in the morning. Continue for 2-3 months and then get off of it.

There are many books written just on gut immunity. I like to address gut immunity using l-glutamine, colostrum, Immunoglobulins, lactoferrin, probiotics and digestive enzymes.

AN IMPORTANT THING TO REMEMBER WHEN DETOXING...

The liver will dump toxins to the small intestines, then to the large intestine to be excreted through the sigmoid colon followed by a bowel movement. In order to not reabsorb these toxins back into your body, one needs to BIND them. I cannot tell you how important it is to use a binder.

Some people use psyllium, bentonite, zeolite, or other clays, but the product I have found on the market that is best tolerated and effective is called "BIND" by *Systemic Formulas*. I would not be without it. Take 3 capsules, twice a day between meals. For people who have mycotoxins and by-products of microbes (yes, microbes crap in us!), this is an essential step.

> No drainage, no detox!

I used liver drainages as well. There is a saying, "Detox without drainage is suicide." I tested for whatever homeopathic extracts my body wanted. Test your body. There so many liver drainages on the market.

H. (HELIOBACTOR) PYLORI

A genetic test is the only test that can accurately diagnose H. Pylori. The breath test and the blood test produce too many false negatives.

My physician touched the upper part of my intestine right under the ribs and I screamed. He said," I think you have H. Pylori". I took a breath test that was negative. I took a blood test where only IgA was positive. The results were inconclusive. So I did an experiment with Gum Mastica and Gastromycin to see if any symptoms of H.Pylori would occur.

Gum Mastica starts the process of killing and releasing H.Pylori while Bismuth in the supplement, Gastromycin, cleans it up from the stomach lining. H. Pylori likes to hang on. If you have a serious ulcer from H. Pylori, please visit a Functional Medicine doctor.

Start with two Gum Mastica in the morning on an empty stomach and two at night, on an empty stomach for 2-3 months. At first you may get a pain in the pit of your stomach after taking two Gum Mastica, but Gastromycin will stop the pain while killing the H. Pylori that are clinging to the stomach wall.

- Take Gastromycin 4 caps with meals, twice a day.

Bismuth, is a necessary but a toxic substance that you will use only for two weeks. Pepto-Bismol has bismuth in it. Some people take Pepto-Bismol because they don't tolerate Gastromycin.

If the pain in the upper part of your stomach goes away, then the bismuth is killing the H. Pylori that is notorious for clinging to the stomach wall. I did not take any antibiotics at all.

There are individuals who eat fermented foods, whether bought or home-made, to address SIBO (Small Intestinal Bacteria Overload). I never felt that fermented vegetables helped me, although I eat raw sauerkraut.

CHAPTER 3
LIVER SUPPORT

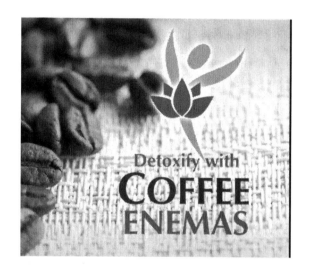

YOU MAY DO COFFEE ENEMAS IF YOU ARE A CBS UPREGULATOR

You may **not** do coffee enemas if you have Crohn's Disease. When I think of liver support, coffee enemas are a priority. From the day I learned I had MCS, I bought *"Wellness Against All Odds,"* by Sherry Rogers, M.D. I did a coffee enema once a day.

Most people are turned off at the thought of any type of enema, never mind coffee enemas. Did you know that coffee enemas have been used for many years? In fact, they were included in the Merck Manual up until 1977.

When detoxifying, toxins are broken down that can make you ill, nauseous, achy and create a feeling of being toxic. With coffee enemas, you are able to eliminate the toxic waste faster. In my view, you are no longer backed-up.

➤ How does a coffee enema work?

The caffeine contained in the coffee circulates via hemorrhoidal veins in the rectum into the enterohepatic system, where it goes directly to the liver via the portal vein.

The portal vein then forces the toxic bile to be eliminated in the gut. The caffeine stimulates the production of glutathione-S-transferase, which is important in making glutathione. Glutathione is a main conjugator for Phase II detoxification which I will now describe in greater detail.

> There are 2 Phases of Detoxification.

Phase I and Phase II. Most people who are chemically sensitive have fast Phase I and normal or slow Phase II. When Phase I is fast, it produces a chemical like formaldehyde many times more toxic than the original compound. Phase II is supported by glutathione. It takes the toxic element from Phase I and adds (conjugates) another molecule which renders the toxin less toxic. When toxic bile is released from the liver into the intestines, wouldn't it be great to bind the toxic sludge? Of course, use your BIND. If you are allergic to BIND, substitute activated charcoal, clay, or zeolite.

Did you know that if you are allergic to coffee, you can still do coffee enemas? Dr. Sherry Rogers sure did! Some people have told me that they do not like the smell. Well, buy an electric burner and brew the coffee outdoors.

If you have tried doing a coffee enema in the past and became sick or were "buzzed" from the caffeine, my modified coffee enema approach will eliminate the caffeinated high.

I have found that most people are able to do coffee enemas successfully using my modified coffee enema instructions.

I do mine every morning!

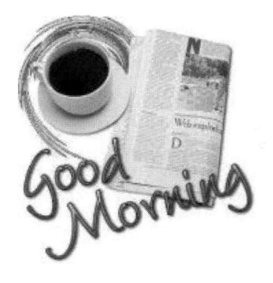

It is important to use coffee made especially for enemas. The ideal coffee is organic light air roasted beans. Air roasted coffee offers a toxin free and mold free bean because it is not processed in a drum. Fire/drum roasting can leave a toxic residue on the bean. Purelifeenema.com offers three types of air roasted beans for enemas …Ultra Light Roast, Light Roast and Medium Roast. Their beans are not only USDA Certified 100% Organic, but are certified organic by a second party as well, The Oregon Tilt. The lighter the roast, the more caffeine the coffee has. If trying an enema for the first time, I recommend the medium roast. For those who have been doing enemas for a long time try the Ultra Light Roast. For those who want a good deal of caffeine but not a blast go for the light roasted. Hey! Experiment! Bulletproof coffee is drum roasted and is not the best coffee for enema therapy. There is SA Wilson's organic coffee that is ground and looks like a yellow grainy powder. It is too strong for the chronically ill. The caffeine content is too high. I have tried this coffee and found that it arrived with a rancid smell probably from being stored in a facility for a while. If you are using it and love it then continue to do so. I am giving you the best information I know as of this date.

What type of enema equipment should I use?

My recommendation is the stainless steel enema bucket kit by purelifeenema.com because it is not made in China or

India but safely made in the USA using clean, inspected USA 304 grade stainless steel, for medical purposes". It never rusts and is easy to clean. They offer a glass enema bucket I use because I have a sensitivity to nickel and I want to see the coffee flowing down the bucket. Nothing can beat the purity of non-toxic glass! I recommend it for the chemically sensitive. Pure Life offers a silicone enema bag far superior to the red latex drugstore enema bag. You can fold it up for easy travel. I recommend browsing www.purelifeenema.com to view everything they offer. Don't miss the enema tubing cleaning brush as coffee stains silicone tubing. If you have questions ask for Susan. She is highly educated in enemas and more. She has been my go to gal.

MODIFIED COFFEE ENEMA
FOR PEOPLE WITH CHRONIC ILLNESS

What You Will Need: A Checklist

- ✓ BIND
- ✓ Magnesium Chloride Solution.
- ✓ Organic Coffee (except Cafe Altura brand).
- ✓ Stainless steel or glass enema bucket kit.
- ✓ Ceramic or glass pot (not stainless steel) to make the coffee in.
- ✓ Stainless steel small mesh strainer.
- ✓ Bodyceuticals Calendula Salve or Unpetroleum Jelly.
- ✓ Disposable Nitrile –Latex-free gloves - sold at any Walgreens.
- ✓ A bathroom toilet stepstool. Sold at Amazon.com

Preparing your Body

- ✓ Take B.I.N.D. 30 minutes before enema
- ✓ To begin, take 1 tablespoon of Magnesium Chloride Solution in 6-8 oz. water.
- ✓ This will relax muscle tissue to ensure ease of release.

✓ Make sure to eat lightly so that you do not become weak. Some people prefer to have a bowel movement before doing the coffee enema. This was not possible for me. I did it when I wanted.

Brewing the Coffee

You will be brewing 4 cups of coffee solution which will be divided into 2 cups used at a time. A complete coffee enema is 2 cups inserted and released followed by an additional 2 cups to be inserted and released.

- Let 2 cups of water come to a boil.

- Add 3 level tablespoons of organic coffee and stir the mixture.

- Lower temperature to a low boil and simmer for 20 minutes.

- Remove from the stove.

- Add 2 cups of cold water to the coffee

- You will now have 4 cups of coffee at approximately lukewarm temperature ready for immediate use. If it is still too hot, add a few ice cubes or wait till it cools.

- Pour coffee through the strainer from the pot and fill it to two cups

- Take the Pyrex cup filled with the 2 cups of coffee solution and bring it to your bathroom.

- Assemble the bucket and tubing and rectal tip.

- Remember to <u>close the clamp</u> on the enema tubing first, or you may end up cleaning up a coffee spill on your bathroom floor! (Yes, I've had that happen too many times!)

- Pour the two cups of coffee from the glass Pyrex measuring cup into the bucket.

- Using the hook that came with your enema kit, hang it from a towel bar in your bathroom.

- If the diameter of the hook that comes with the kit is too small, improvise and purchase a large S hook in your local hardware store. The enema needs to be hung in a low position. Do not hang it from a shower rod or shower head.

- Place the enema bucket on a hook hanging from a towel rack with the 2 cups of coffee in it.

- Place a towel on the floor. (I use a brown one. LOL!)

- Place the Calendula Salve or Unpetroleum Jelly close to you.

You are now ready to do it!

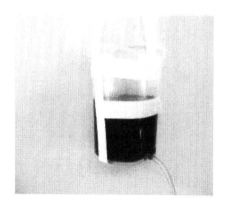

THE 6 STEP MODIFIED COFFEE ENEMA TECHNIQUE

1. Lubricate
2. Insert
3. Hold
4. Release
5. Massage
6. Disinfect

The First Half (500 ml or 2 cups)

Let enough coffee solution flow out of the enema bucket to create a free flow without air bubbles going into the rectum. You can use the toilet bowl to dump it. Then add more water warm to the bucket so it is exactly 2 cups to account for the coffee solution that was previously dumped out.

Step 1. Lubricate

- Pick up the rectal tip of the enema tubing and lubricate it with the Calendula salve or Unpetroleum Jelly. [Do not use "Preparation H" as it contains Mercury, "Vaseline" or "KY-Jelly," because both contain petroleum.]

Step 2. Insert

- Lying on your left side, insert the rectal enema tip as far as it can go into the rectum.

- Unclamp the tubing letting a little coffee solution in but not too much to cause cramping. Take the enema tip out of your rectum each time and wait several seconds until the urge to go is gone.

- Insert again and again, till coffee solution is almost gone. Some coffee will remain behind in the bucket due to its design.

Step 3. Hold

- You may need to hold the tube or tip so that it doesn't slip from your anus.

- Soon you will teach your body to retain the coffee solution long enough to be effective.

➢ The goal is to hold 2 cups of coffee solution for 10-15 minutes.

Fifteen minutes is preferred. It is how long you hold it that matters the most rather than the quantity of coffee you insert. In the beginning it feels like a tall order.

➢ Be patient! Practice makes perfect.

Step 4. Release

Make sure your toilet stepstool is in place. After 15 minutes, release the coffee into the toilet. I can't send you photos of this, but I pick up the toilet seat and kneel on the rim, feet flat in a squat. I then release the enema solution. Remember, I didn't weigh a lot when I first started doing coffee enemas. So, it was easy.

Some time ago, when I was in Paris, France, with a boyfriend, I was on the street looking for a bathroom. I entered a lavatory. To my surprise, I found what looked like a hole in the ground. I ran out completely startled.

The toilet bowl is missing," I shouted. No, people told us that some bathrooms outside are designed so you can squat and go!

Do go and buy a footstool. You can find them online, at Amazon.com. It is essential for proper evacuation!

Step 5. Rectal Massage

This is the most important step not to be ignored. You must do it! If you leave it out you are likely to get sick. In fact, if you don't do this step then don't do a coffee enema. It is called the rectal massage. Read carefully as this step is often misunderstood. Your rectum is inside of your body. Your anus is the opening.

- Release as much coffee solution as you can until you can't release any further.

- Put on your disposable Nitrile glove

- Using your index finger, insert it into your rectum (where you inserted the enema tip) up to your knuckles.

- Begin to massage or tickle the mucous membrane walls in the rectum long enough to cause peristalsis.

More toxic crap will come out of you. Please forgive the language, but few people get this right. I have never met anyone who didn't need to use this technique. So, if you are wired you have skipped this step. Is it messy? Yes. Is it worth doing? Darn right!

Folks have told me, "Oh My God, I didn't think it was possible to have anything left in me." I remind them "Just when you think you have finished, go back and massage again."

Step 6. Disinfect

- Please be sure to wash your hands thoroughly. Use a nailbrush to scrub under your fingernails and cuticles.
- Make it a habit to not place your fingers in your mouth.
- Wash the silicone tubing using an 8 ounce squirt jar filled with liquid soap of your choice.
- Rinse it with plain water.
- Hang to dry. You are ready to move on.

The Second Half (500 ml or 2 Cups)

- Now you are ready to do the 2nd half of the coffee enema.
- Check the temperature of the 2 remaining cups of coffee in the pot.
- It it's too cold, heat it to the desired temperature.

Repeat Step 1, 2, 3, 4, 5 and 6

- Again, clean the silicone tubing using an 8 ounce squirt bottle filled with a liquid soap of your choice. Squirt the soap into both ends of the tubing. Then fill the tubing with water.

- Let the tubing filled with soapy water sit for a few minutes and rinse well. Hang the tubing to dry. Clean your toilet bowl using a brush and disinfectant of your choice.

- After a few days, you will get the hang of it. You will begin to see and SMELL the chemicals being released. That's right.

➢ Congratulations! You just completed your first proper coffee enema! You are a Brave Soul!

You will be one of the fortunate ones who will get well fast and suffer minimally. You now have an important tool to use for detoxification and healing.

CASTOR OIL PACKS

Castor oil packs have been used for many conditions including liver problems. Castor oil when heated on wool or cotton flannel, acts as a counter irritant. It irritates the skin surface, causing dilation of the vessels and recruitment of immune cells to the area under the pack.

For convenience buy a castor oil kit. It will come with the wool or cotton flannel, whichever you prefer. Sometimes the castor oil comes with the kit, if not purchase it separately. Do not reuse the flannel cloth. Years ago you were told to refrigerate it and use over and over again. This will cause the chemicals from the used flannel to reenter your body.

> How to Use a Castor Oil Pack

Place the flannel cloth to fit over the liver. Cut a piece of plastic or plastic wrap one to two inches larger than the flannel cloth. Soak the flannel cloth in gently heated castor oil. Squeeze some liquid out.

Prepare the surface where you will be lying. Place a large plastic sheet and an old towel over the surface to prevent staining. Lie down on the towel and place the oil-soaked flannel over your liver. Place fitted plastic piece over the flannel cloth. Apply a hot water bottle over the area. You can cover with another towel.

Rest for one to two hours. Wash your body with a solution of three tablespoons baking soda to one quart water to rinse off the oil, or you will get a rash.

LIVER FLUSH

I do not recommend a liver flush at this time. It is too hard on your adrenals. Yes, I know people swear by them, but many energy practitioners and I do not.

DRY SKIN BRUSHING

Aids the body in detoxification, of course the exfoliation part is easy to understand. As for detoxing, dry skin brushing is similar to massage. The light pressure against your skin and the direction in which you brush helps move lymph fluid into the lymph nodes so this waste can be eliminated.

Dry skin brushing boosts circulation, delivering oxygenated blood to the skin and other organs, which helps them do their jobs better.

So, How Do You Dry Skin Brush?

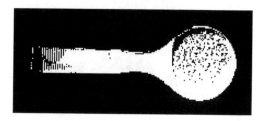

- First you need a proper brush which you can purchase at most health food stores. Look for firm bristles vegetable-derived. A long handle is required for those hard to reach areas such as your back.

- Because dry brushing energizes and stimulates the body, most practitioners suggest doing it in the morning before you shower, but you can do it any time of the day you prefer.

- Using long, upward strokes, start brushing your skin at your feet and work up your legs one at a time.

- Then move up your mid-section (front and back) and across your chest.

- Finish up your arms toward your armpits.

- Some people say the detox and circulatory boost helps with digestive issues and skin problems such as acne.

CHAPTER 4
EMF

ELECTROMAGNETIC FIELD SENSITIVITY SUPPORT

A 21ST CENTURY TROJAN HORSE

Electromagnetic Field Sensitivity or EMF is an adverse reactivity of the body to electric and magnetic stimuli.

The typical 21st Century home has many devices which employ microwave technology. These include, microwave ovens, mobile phones and iPads, digital cordless phones, Wi-Fi, wireless internet connectors, Bluetooth wireless devices, burglar alarms with microwave detectors, and digital cordless baby monitors.

In 2016, the European Environmental Agency, Europe's top environmental watchdog responded to the growing evidence by calling for immediate action to reduce exposure to radiation from Wi-Fi and mobile phones -suggesting that the delay could lead to a health crisis similar to those associated with asbestos, smoking and lead in gasoline.

In Germany, the government is advising its citizens to use wired internet connections whenever possible, instead of Wi-Fi and landlines instead of mobile phones.

In Sweden, recognition of the dangers is already well-developed. Electro-sensitivity is recognized as a disability. They are so progressive, unlike the USA, where ES is not recognized as a disabling condition.

A frightening new 2017 study says that allowing a baby to play on an iPad might lead to speech delays.

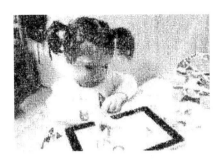

A presentation of the Academic Societies Meeting, revealed startling findings, (CNN by Kelly Wallace). The study found that the more time children between the ages of six months and two years spent using handheld screens such as smart phone tablets and electronic games, the more likely they were to develop speech delays.

"I believe it's the first study to examine mobile media devices and communication delay in children," said Dr. Catherine Birken, the study's senior investigator, a Pediatrician and scientist at the Hospital for Sick Children in Toronto, Ontario. It really shines a light on the issue. Nine hundred children were involved in the study.

Nearly 90% of children under age 2 have used a mobile device, an increase from just 10% in 2011, according to a 2013 study by Common Sense Media Technology.

What is difficult about avoiding electromagnetic fields is that they are invisible. Many people are in denial regarding EMF's harmfulness because of this. It is so easy to have Wi-Fi, and keep your phone close by.

For the Chemically Sensitive, you have to go cold turkey for 7-8 weeks. I am serious. Those who are electromagnetically hypersensitive, there is no choice.

- The Symptoms are:
  - Numbness and tingling in the extremities
  - Seizures
  - Impaired cognition
  - Severe migraine headaches,
  - Vomiting
  - Shaking
  - Feeling as though you were electrocuted

How does one live in the
21st Century with
this kind of sensitivity?

Almost Impossible!

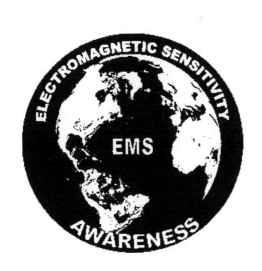

CHAPTER 5
THE SAUNA PROGRAM

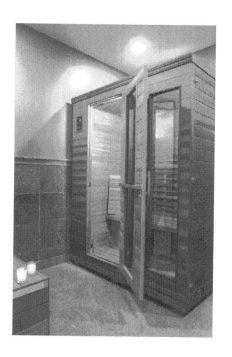

- You may sauna if you are a CBS Upregulator. Eliminate the glutathione. You may sauna even if you are EMF sensitive by heating the sauna beforehand and unplugging the unit.

Today, there are many different types of sauna. High dry heat, far infrared, and ozone saunas are the most commonly known. I used a high heat cloth sauna from Fred Nelson. (No longer with us). It is no longer available. I started at the Environmental Health Center in Dallas, with William Rea, M.D. as my doctor. If you have chemical sensitivity to wood, and most likely you do, I would only consider finding a used, out gassed sauna. Eighteen years ago, I couldn't safely go into any wooden sauna except the tiled sauna at Dr. Rea's clinic and my cloth sauna.

- Rule of Thumb...

If you sauna three or more times a week, a weekly fasting blood test is in order. You can obtain a prescription from your doctor and take it to your nearest lab.

The chemically sensitive person usually has low ferritin levels. My ferritin level was 2 and Dr. Rea still advised me to sauna. Ideally it should be 15 but who has a ferritin level of 15 when they are that sick and malnourished. Many women have a ferritin level of 6-12.

- ✓ Take a multivitamin/multi-mineral with iron if your ferritin levels are low. I couldn't tolerate iron and Dr. Rea still advised me to sauna. You do what you have to do.

- ✓ Some say cook in a cast iron pan for iron. That is what I do. Men and post- menopausal women do not need to take the additional iron supplement.

- ➢ If at any point, you are uncomfortable or woozy in the sauna, "Get Out!"

  - Try to eat one hour before beginning sauna.

  - If you eat a big breakfast followed by a sauna, you might vomit.

  - If you are taking prescription medications, take them after your sauna so you won't sweat them out.

- ➢ Your goal is to teach the body to sweat and use sauna as a chelator of toxic chemicals.

Approximately 20% of toxins will come out of your skin through sweating and outgassing. Approximately 80% of toxins will be excreted through the liver and kidneys dumping into the colon and into the bladder to be excreted as urine and fecal matter.

Sauna transforms fat soluble chemicals into water soluble chemicals ready for excretion via the detox organs- namely the liver, kidney and skin.

The period of time one stays in the sauna varies from individual to individual. A person may remain comfortably in the sauna for only 10 minutes, while another person may stay for 20 minutes. Your level of health will determine the duration of your sauna session.

When you have reached 30 minutes, you may try another round later the same day. When beginning, it is best to wait several hours before a second- round of sauna.

Preparation for Sauna

- Take your weight.
- Exercise if you can. If you have Chronic Fatigue, do not exercise beforehand.
- In 6 oz. of water, add:
- ½ teaspoon of Tri-salts (Ecological Formulas).
- 1/8 teaspoon of salt.
- 1 teaspoon Magnesium Chloride (ARG).
- 200 mg. buffered Vitamin C.
- 500 mg. Liposomal Glutathione (do not take if you are a CBS++).
- ½ tsp. Selenium Selenite (ARG) or selenium methionine. (Whatever you can tolerate)

- You can take a Niacin supplement used to vasodilate your blood vessels. I could not tolerate it. If you do want to try niacin then start with 25mgs.

Temperature Setting

- High Heat: No more than 150 degrees. Yes, I know people go higher, but do not.
- Infrared, can be as low as 110 degrees.

What to wear and bring with you:

- Several large glasses with 12 oz. of clean water for each 15 minutes in the sauna. (No plastic bottles).
- You can sauna naked or wear a tee shirt and shorts.
- A wash cloth or small towel to dry up every bead of sweat. We do not want any reabsorption.
- A towel to sit on.

The key to sauna is to find a balance between "downloading" (I like this computer tech term!) chemicals from fatty tissue, chelating them, and excreting them without adding to your existing load.

After the Sauna...

Shower and Scrub: Immediately after the sauna, take a shower, making sure to use a washcloth to scrub down your body.

After Sauna Supplements...

It's not over till it's over, so remember to take these supplements after each sauna session.

- ½ tsp/ Tri-salts dissolved in water.
- 1/8 tsp salt.
- Multivitamin/multi-mineral caps with or without iron.3 Tablespoons of olive oil or coconut oil; or any tolerated oil is OK.
- 1 Tablespoon of psyllium.
- Check your weight. If you weigh less than you did before sauna, you are dehydrated and need to drink another glass of water.

About the Process

If you need to proceed more slowly, or you are able to proceed faster than this program suggests, please do so. You are in charge of your body. Remember, when trying out this new sauna program, "Be Confident." It will all work out. It is your personal best that is the goal- not what your friends can do.

Ozone Saunas are different. They combine steam with ozone. Your head will be extended out of the chamber. People with reactive airways do not do well with ozone.

If you are considering one, it's a good idea to research and try an ozone sauna session in a certified practitioner's office before buying the equipment needed to set it up at home. I did not use an ozone sauna till 2010. My experience using this type of sauna was exhilarating. Ozone doesn't bother me when used correctly, in a well ventilated room. There are rectal/vaginal ozone suppositories I use that are sold at Promolife.com. They come in a choice of base oils.

EXAMPLE OF A 7-WEEK SAUNA PROGRAM

Your sauna program can last from seven weeks to a seven week program every six months depending on your degree of toxicity. I was emaciated. I was all bones, allergic to everything, especially food. If you are like me, you are going to have to start slowly. Do not take Niacin. Do not be concerned if you do not sweat right away. You probably will not. Your sauna schedule might look like this:

WEEK 1:

Day One: 5-10 minutes in sauna
Day Two: 10 minutes
Day Three: 10 minutes
Day Four: 15 minutes
Day Five: 15 minutes

Day Six: 15 minutes
Day Seven: 15 minutes

WEEK 2:

Day One: 20 minutes
Day Two: 20 minutes
Day Three: 20 minutes
Day Four: 20 minutes
Day Five: 20 minutes
Day Six: 20 minutes
Day Seven: 20 minutes

WEEK 3

Try to increase your sauna time by 5 minutes to 25 minutes daily.

WEEK 4

Again increase your sauna time by 5 minutes to 30 minutes daily. I had the hardest time increasing it. I could never get past 20 minutes for 7 weeks. One more time! Do your personal best.

WEEK 5-7

Maintain your 30 minutes sauna time or stay at your longest comfortable time.

EXAMPLE OF A SAUNA PROGRAM FOR A HEALTHIER PERSON

I call the person with a normal body weight "Healthier". She or he appears to be someone who is not ill, but has high levels of toxic chemicals in their body. They may suffer from chronic fatigue. They may be able to eat many foods.

If you are a healthier, here's what your sauna schedule might look like.

You can add 25mgs.-75mgs. of niacin as you exercise. You will have a red flush all over your body. If you can tolerate niacin, use it. It dilates the blood vessels which makes for a deeper detoxification.

WEEK 1
Day One: 20 minutes
Day Two: 20 minutes
Day Three: 25 minutes
Day Four: 30 minutes
Day Five: 30 minutes
Day Six: 35 minutes
Day Seven: 35 minutes

WEEK 2:

You may be ready for two rounds of 30 minutes daily
Day One: AM 30 minutes; PM 30 minutes
Day Two: AM: 30 minutes; PM: 30 minutes
Continue to Day 7

<u>WEEK 3-7</u>

Two 45 minute rounds daily

SAUNA MAINTENANCE SCHEDULE

The schedules above are only examples. You will determine your sauna time. After 7 weeks of the 7 Day sauna detoxification program, you may go on a maintenance program. In 6 months, some people feel the need to undergo, once again, the 7-day intensive two rounds of a sauna detoxification program.

I've been told that there is a barrier to break in sauna. Your body begins to experience the hot air as cool. I have never broken that barrier. I am not able to stay in a high heat or infrared sauna that long.

There is disagreement in the world about how much to sauna. Some experts believe fully in the L. Ron Hubbard approach in rounds and rounds of sauna in one day for a period of weeks, while others advise doing sauna only 2-3 times weekly at best. Nevertheless, all agree that nutrients are essential.

Women who are chemically sensitive take longer to break out in a sweat. Do not worry, it will happen.

Congratulations!
You have learned how to Sauna!

CHAPTER 6
PEARLS

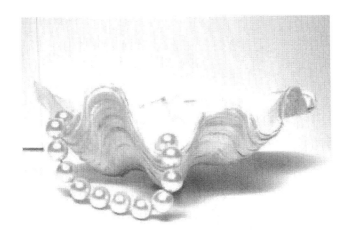

First Pearl – No ALA...

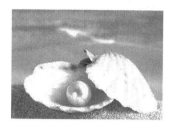

Never use the supplement Alpha Lipoic Acid in the beginning of your detoxification. Look at your supplements, especially your multivitamins and multi-minerals. If it even has 10-20mgs you may not take it. Take this advice very seriously. In my past I took 600mgs a day of ALA, as I was following a practitioner's program. (I will not mention who). I started having suicidal ideation, severe insomnia, and trembling. I stuck with this program for some time. I wasted time and unnecessary suffering. ALA is not just an antioxidant, it is a brain chelator for heavy metals, especially mercury. According to Andy Cutler, I was taking huge amounts of ALA which is contraindicated. I agree. ALA penetrates the blood brain barrier which causes heavy metals like mercury to come out of the brain. Unless you are on an appropriate chelation program the metals will just recirculate back to the brain causing many negative symptoms which happened in my case.

This is a problem because the chemically sensitive in the beginning of detoxification are not ready to chelate metal from their brain.

Instead of starting with nutrition and cleansing the ALA is now chelating your brain. Who would race straight to chelation of the brain?

Why do alternative practitioners still recommend ALA if it is not part of a chelation program? Your guess is as good as mine. I told you in my introduction I would be giving you pearls of information. I delivered. Do not use ALA under any circumstances unless under the care of a practitioner who specializes in brain chelation.

If a practitioner is still doing IV chelation walk away. Every chelator can be taken orally or rectally. It is a safety concern to have IV chelation.

Second Pearl – MarCons

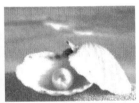

A MarCons nasal swab test is necessary for the chemically sensitive even if you do not have sinus issues. Ask your doctor, "What is a MarCons test? She/he will have no idea. It can be purchased online for $85.00. I used Microbiology DX to test for MarCons. The pricing for the Nares Bacterial Culture includes MarCons and other bacterial pathogens is $85.00.

The request form states that a healthcare practitioner's referral is required, but you can indicate on the order that the results be sent to your home. If it isn't approved, you can ask your healthcare provider to assist in ordering the product. You may be teaching her/him something new!

If you can't use a computer, the telephone number is 718-276-4957. They are located in Bedford, MA.

MarCons stands for "Multiple Antibiotic Resistant Coagulase Negative Staphylococcus." How's that for a mouthful! Before taking the test look up the MarCons nasal swap test demo on You Tube. Boy! That was good advice. You must do the same otherwise the nasal stick will not go deep enough into the sinuses to have an accurate diagnosis. I did it, be brave you can too!

If your MarCons test is positive you can work with an experienced practitioner specializing in MarCons. I'm oversimplifying but basically you will be given an antibiotic spray called BEG spray. I chose a more natural approach using a combination of water, salt, xylitol and Tri-salts.

- ➢ Dr. Deitrich Klinghardt has a Formula Using:
    - 4 cups tepid H2O (not too hot, not too cold)
    - 1 tablespoon Himalayan salt
    - 1 tablespoon Kal brand xylitol because it is a fine powder, otherwise use any other brand.
    - 1 tablespoon Tri-salts (he uses baking soda)
    - Using a glass jar, shake the above ingredients until the mixture is dissolved. Save for later use.

I use the SinuPulse Elite to flush out my sinuses using Dr. Klinghardt's recipe. It is an advanced Nasal Sinus Irrigation System recommended by leading ENTs, Allergists and Pediatricians. It is designed and engineered in Switzerland. It is a pulsatile device. The gentle smooth pulsing of this solution through a customized tip cleanses the nose and sinuses of allergens, dust, dirt and pollens, and actually helps to enhance ciliary flow.

The SinuPulse Elite is beneficial for sinus-related snoring and environmental conditions including pollution, smoke, smog, or chemical exposure. Dr. Robert Iver, author of the best-selling book, "Sinus Survival," wrote, "I recommend the SinuPulse, which is the premiere state-of-the-art irrigation device and the only one capable of delivering a moisturizing, mist spray or more through therapeutic measures in completely eliminating a sinus infection and treating sinusitis. It can help quickly and dramatically."

I purchased mine at Amazon.com. I tested MarCons negative after two months of Dr. Klinghardt's formula and using SinuPulse Elite. That is amazing! And I avoided antibiotics. I am aware that people use neti pots. I do not recommend them.

MarCons and other infections will return if a person has a deviated septum. Sometimes you can see a crookedness in the nose. If you don't know whether you have a deviated septum, ask your practitioner. If it is not corrected by surgery, then the above nasal wash should be used daily.

The Nasopure nasal wash bottle is an affordable way to wash out your sinuses and can be used when travelling. It is assembled by adults with disabilities, BPA free plastic, is made in Missouri, and is USA and FDA registered. It can be purchased at Walgreens.

Third Pearl – Tudca

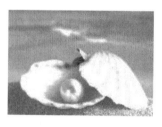

Years ago, I came across a bodybuilder who used steroids. Did you know that his liver enzymes were elevated from steroids? ALT, -alamine transanudase +AST – aspartate transaminase are enzymes in the liver as well as other organs in the body.

He would take a supplement called Tudca to lower the enzyme level in order to remain on steroids. Tudca worked and is well known to body builders.

In the chronically ill individual, liver enzymes are often high. I met a young teenager at the Dallas Environmental

Health Center who had elevated liver enzymes that would not come down despite treatment. Her mother secretly came to my apartment one night and asked me how her daughter should do a coffee enema.

Had it been today, I would have recommended Tudca immediately. Nevertheless, the coffee enema accomplished the goal of lowering her liver enzyme level.

Fourth Pearl – Hormetic Stress

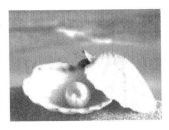

I hear the term hormetic stress used in recovery for chronic illnesses. Hormetic stress is when you apply a good source of stress to the body in order for it to become stronger. Examples in this book are sauna, ozone sauna, colon cleanse, coffee enemas, LED Zyto or Asyra treatments, mini-trampoline and antioxidants. I advise a person with chronic fatigue or adrenal fatigue to use the above treatments. Chronic fatigue and adrenal fatigue overlap in so many areas.

If a chronically ill person uses cold water after the end of their shower it will benefit the adrenal glands. It seems counterintuitive, but it works. When I first heard of the use of cold to help me in recovery I snapped at my friend saying, "My adrenal glands have enough stress." He kindly said do it for thirty seconds. I continue to do it today... a little longer now! Hard training aerobic workouts are good hormetic stress for healthy people but would not be good hormetic stress for chronically ill people.

Also the idea of using low dose chemical exposure for MCS people would be bad hormetic stress. It doesn't work. So, hormetic stress is just not exercise and fasting for healthier people, it can be done with the chronically ill as well. By the way, if you can't jump on the mini-trampoline, have someone jump for you while you sit on it. It will be just as effective, especially if you are in a wheel chair. When I was very ill a friend lent me her mini-trampoline. I jumped for twenty minutes and vomited for forty eight hours. Now that was too much hormetic stress. I couldn't look at a trampoline for months. I had loathed it. Five minutes would have been sufficient. Each person will have her/his own balance of hormetic stress. It is a balancing act. If you lightly exercise and end up in bed for two days, then it is bad hormetic stress. In another chronically ill person it may be good. You will find your balance of good and bad hormetic stress.

Fifth Pearl – Naltrexone

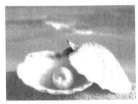

Naltrexone is a drug used in the treatment of addiction. It is prescribed at 150mgs. It is now being used for the chronically ill at 4.5mgs. It is an immune booster. Your physician will have to give you a prescription as well as directions. Naltrexone made a big difference in lowering my sensitivities to chemicals. I stopped taking it for one month and went back on because I was becoming more chemically sensitive. To this day I am on 4.5mgs of naltrexone.

CHAPTER 7
ORAL SUPPLEMENTS

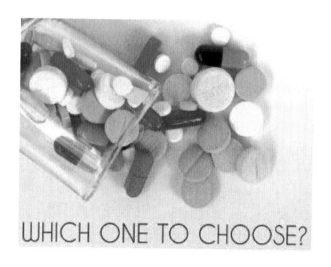

WHICH ONE TO CHOOSE?

➢ The supplements discussed here are only suggested supplements. If you are taking others and are doing well, and you have been tested, continue to take them.

➢ If you are a CBS Upregulator, no sulfur containing or promoting supplements should be taken as mentioned in Chapter One.

Vitamin C: Chemically sensitive people do better when Vitamin C is buffered. It can be from tapioca, corn, or cassava. Ideally, the dose is to bowel tolerance, but you will proceed slowly. Start with 500-1,000 mg of Vitamin C daily and work up to 800mgs every other day. Capsules are more convenient. If you can tolerate liposomal Vitamin C which is more bioavailable then it is preferred. Follow label directions. Vitamin C helps with free radical damage occurring to the mitochondria in fast Phase I of detoxification. It's an antioxidant and anti-inflammatory.

B-Complex: Vitamin B is one of the least tolerated vitamins for the chemically sensitive. However, it is very important. B1, B2, B3, B5 all help in fast Phase I of detoxification. One, once a day.

Hydroxyl B12: Sublingual or intramuscular injection. Take one lozenge sublingually, one to two times daily.

Multivitamin/Multi-mineral: Start with one daily, with Iron if you are doing sauna. (see Sauna section)

L-Glutamine: heals a leaky gut. Follow directions on label.

Liposomal Glutathione: 500-1,000 mg once daily. Liposomal glutathione is more bioavailable. Do not use reduced glutathione in capsules.

5-Methyltetrahydrofolate: 5-MTHF – start with 5 mgs.

Magnesium Citrate or Glycinate: till bowel tolerance.

Magnesium Chloride solution: Start with 1/2 teaspoon in 6 oz. water.

Tudca: Liver support; One daily

Candi-Pro: 2 caps twice daily on an empty stomach. Contains Colostrum, Immunoglobulins lactoferrin, and probiotics. It is an immune booster as well as a support for Candida overgrowth

B.I.N.D: Binder of toxins in the digestive tract, 3 capsules 2x daily.

Omega 3 Fish Oil: 1 capsule every other day. Restores brain health.

Probiotics: Aides in microbial overgrowth to strengthen the immune system. Add probiotic you can tolerate. Make sure it includes lactobacillus rhamnosus. It helps with anxiety.

Pancreatic Enzymes: Before or between meals. Help with digestion and inflammation.

Digestive enzymes: Use before any meal. Helps with digestion. Use as many as it takes to digest. Usually 1-5 enzymes.

L-citrulline: to reduce ammonia. Once daily between meals.

Tri-salts: See Sauna section; to help keep alkalinize take 1/2 teaspoon in 4 oz. water before bedtime.

Organic coconut oil.

Organic olive oil.

Licorice or DGL: Once a day for adrenal support.

Lymph drainage: for lymph support.

Kidney drainage: for kidney support.

Immune care Candigest Plus Capsules: to kill Candida species without die off. Helps the immune system. Take one-two capsules before breakfast and one-two capsules at bedtime with warm water.

Vitamin D: full spectrum. Strengthens the immune system.

Lugol's Iodine: Start with one drop. Helps with thyroid function.

Zinc Glyconate: 1 capsule or 1 sublingual lozenge daily. Best absorbable form. It protects the liver from chemical damage.

Gum Mastica: 1-2 capsules first thing in the morning and 1-2 capsules at bedtime. Gastromycin: 4 capsules twice a day with meals for two weeks. (While taking Mastica).

Homeopathic Histamine: 8-drops as needed for a reaction.

Quercetin: is a bioflavonoid that is good to take in a reaction along with Vitamin C.

Gaba: an amino acid that acts as a neurotransmitter in the central nervous system. Gaba can be taken to calm the body because it inhibits neuron activity from firing.

Niacin: start with 25 mgs. When you sauna; if tolerated. It is needed for proper circulation and healthy skin.

Taurine: 500 mg once daily. It is a building block for all the other amino acids as well as the component of bile, which is needed in the digestion of fats. Taurine has a protective effect on the brain. It is used to treat anxiety and seizures.

Selenium: 200 mcg a day. It inhibits the oxidation of lipids (fats) as a component of the enzyme glutathione peroxidase.

Grapeseed Extract: 50-100 mg a day. Anti-inflammatory, anti-microbial, and antioxidant.

Yucca: 500 mg twice a day. It is anti-inflammatory and aides in digestion. It aides in ammonia support.

Cherry fruit extract: Take 2 capsules three times daily. It aides in ammonia support in CBS Upregulators.

COQ10 and L- carnitine: There is a deficiency in CBS Upregulators. Dosage depends on person. They help to facilitate the production of ATP.

Activated Charcoal: to aide in ammonia absorption.

Royal Jelly: It contains Biopterin which aides in ammonia support for CBS Upregulators.

CHAPTER 8
RECTAL USE OF SUPPLEMENTS

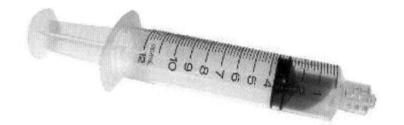

In 1977, I formulated a rectal liquid nutrient called CoRectalVite, which was manufactured by Stephen Levine, PhD, of Allergy Research Group /Nutricology. The supplement is no longer on the market due to FDA regulations. The 100 cc sterile preservative free solution was packaged in a darkened glass bottle. CoRectalVite contained 15grams of Vitamin C, 15 ml of Magnesium Chloride, 2 ml of trace minerals, 2 grams of Taurine, 600 mg Glutathione, B complex, and 2ml of Methyl B12.

This formulation had been given intravenously at the Environmental Health Center in Dallas, Texas. I had been given the IV formula but became allergic to the stainless steel needles and had to discontinue the IV detoxification. I gave it great consideration and decided I would make my own saline and add the detoxing nutrients. I used an enema bag and inserted the nutrients rectally, holding them all day or all night. It was a retention enema.

For years, I have used Vitamin C, magnesium chloride, and glutathione rectally. Today, rectal nutrients are becoming cutting edge.

HOW TO MAKE VITAMIN C FOR RECTAL USE

- Use an unbuffered Vitamin C powder. You can use 100-800 mg.
- Stir in 500 ml of pure drinking water and add a pinch of salt.
- Stir till the powder is dissolved.
- Place the Vitamin C solution directly into your enema bucket. Insert as you would a coffee enema and hold for as long as you can.

HOW TO MAKE RECTAL GLUTATHIONE

The following recipe can be used to make rectal Glutathione which will be equivalent to an IV or IV push.

- Buy, online, 12 cc syringes without a needle, by Monocot. You can purchase a box of 100 for 16.00 on amazon.com.
- Buy Glutathione powder without any fillers.
- Put 500 ml of Glutathione powder and pour into a lidded jar. (A small jam/jelly jar works perfectly).
- Add 12 cc pure drinking water to the powder. Cover and shake till dissolved.
- Draw the glutathione solution into the 12 cc barrel.
- Shake out any bubbles which may have formed. Insert rectally with or without lubrication.

HOW TO MAKE RECTAL SUPPOSITORIES

- Purchase OXO Good Grips No-Spill Silicone Ice Stick Tray for suppositories, on Amazon.com for $16.30.

- You can make 12 suppositories or less at a time

> Vitamin C Recipe:
- Melt, lightly, 2 tsps. Of organic coconut oil till liquid. (Be sure it is not hot).

- Add 1000-8000 mg of Unbuffered Vitamin C powder and stir.

- Pour the mixture into the silicone molds and put in the refrigerator. Take it out when it is hard.

- Insert rectally.

> Glutathione recipe:
- You can add 500 mg of Glutathione powder to make the suppositories using the same method above.

RECTAL SUPPOSITORIES FOR CONSTIPATION IN TODDLERS

My friend, has a 2-year old daughter who had constipation. She asked me for a natural remedy and I shared this recipe for suppositories.

- Purchase OXO silicone mold ice trays from Amazon.com

- Use 1 tsp liquid coconut oil (melted) and mix with 1 teaspoon of cocoa butter.

- Place mold in refrigerator. After 1 hour remove from fridge.

- The suppository should be cut in half for toddlers and inserted rectally.

A HOME CURE FOR HEMORRHOIDS

➢ Never, ever use *Preparation H* for hemorrhoids. The product contains Mercury.

- A home cure is to mix garlic and Witch Hazel into coconut oil. Use a garlic press.

- The ratio is 1 part garlic to 10 parts coconut oil, to 10 drops of Witch Hazel. Stir it up and pour it into OXO silicone molds.

- Place in Refrigerator. Wait till it hardens.

- Insert one suppository rectally at night until cured.

- You can go stronger and use a 1:5 ratio of garlic to coconut oil.

VAGINAL SUPPOSITORIES FOR YEAST OR BACTERIAL INFECTION

- Use OXO silicone mold trays. Starting with the first mold, fill half with organic yogurt.

- Next, open half of a probiotic capsule. Preferably, use one with Lactobacillus Acidophilus plus Bifidus and add it to the yogurt.

- Then, fill to the top with more organic yogurt.

- Freeze it and insert one suppository at night.

- Please use an organic cotton sanitary napkin. Continue for 7-9 days.

WHAT CAN I EXPECT DURING THE DETOXIFICATION PROCESS

➢ Expect Anything and Everything to Happen!

Some people begin to do coffee enemas and sauna and enter a gentle detox. Others do the same and detox with a BANG! So it was for me. Here are some of the things you may experience as you detox. They are described here so that you will be prepared if they occur. By knowing what to expect, you will not be frightened and will persevere. Remember that the process of detoxification can mimic a reaction, however it is never as extreme a reaction as a toxic exposure.

➢ If you want to break a reaction, take:

- 1 Tsp Magnesium Solution
- ½ Tsp Tri-salts
- 2000 mg. Vitamin C.
- Or take Alka Seltzer Gold.
- Or take quercetin with or without nettles.

➢ Numbness, Tingling and Muscle Weakness

After my first sauna, I awakened in the morning with stiffness in the fingers of my right hand. When I tried to bend them, I was in horrific pain. The right side of my body seemed to have been affected. This is common. Also common is numbness and a tingling sensation in the extremities. People have reported detox symptoms occurring on either the right or left side of their bodies. If I tried to support my head with my right hand while lying down, my wrist would give in. While walking, my right ankle would slip out from under me causing me to nearly fall. One morning when I awoke, I felt as though a three-ton elephant was sitting on my chest. The difficulty breathing subsided quickly.

➢ Transient Skin Reactions & "Creepy Crawlies."

- Transient skin reactions are common. Here are some you may experience:
- A burning skin sensation
- Chemical liquid coming out of your nipples
- Acne or dry skin patches resembling eczema
- Dryness of your fingertips especially on your thumb.
- Bleeding knuckles

Also, there were occasions when I felt as if 1000 ants were crawling over my body. Sometimes I would slap my thigh thinking an insect had bitten me. One of my friends reported "seeing spiders" in her room before closing the light at night. This is more common than you'd think.

➤ Anxiety and Panic Attacks

In the past, I suffered from anxiety and panic attacks. Detoxification never intensified them. In fact, anxiety was gone with sauna and rectal nutrients. When you detox the chemicals that caused the attacks, you feel you are beginning to have an attack, but it never comes. This was a tremendous relief for me

➤ Sleep Disturbances

You can expect that your sleep will be disturbed. You may have night sweats. It is vital that you get sufficient sleep. Do what you must to get 8 hours or more of restful sleep. Eight hours of sleep from 10 pm to 6 am is more beneficial than sleeping from 1 am to 9 am. I slept from 9:30 pm to 6:30 am for three months of my detox program. Since most people in a detox awake in the early morning, it's wise to do the same. I now sleep from 11 pm to 8 am.

You will have night sweats, especially in the beginning of sauna. This is a good sign. I would soak the bed with sweat and wash off in the shower at 3:00am because Dr.

Rea told me to. I was such a good student. If you can't do that then at least keep a hand towel to wipe down. You don't want to reabsorb toxins coming out.

- ✓ All electronic and EMF devices must be shut off after 6:00 pm. Do not sleep with a TV on.

- ✓ Close the lights ½ hour before going to sleep. The room should be dark enough that you cannot see your hand close up.

➤ **Fatigue, Nausea, the Munchies and Brain Fog.**

Be prepared for initial fatigue and/or temporary hyperactivity. After two sauna treatments I became very hyperactive. I had to tie my ankles together so I wouldn't get up so many times. No kidding! There will be times when you will feel nauseous when coming out of the sauna. I sometimes vomited if my stomach was too empty. There may also be times, after sauna, when you will eat yourself out of house and home… the major munchies! Don't be alarmed if, after sauna and taking rectal nutrients you experience an hour or so of intense "brain fog," it will pass. Remember, stay calm and never panic. It's all part of the process.

Find other people with MCS
who will become your good friends.
Go through this program together!

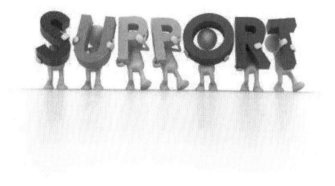

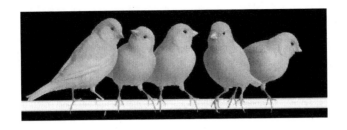

To all of you out there in "Detox City,

I Wish You Good Fortune
on Your Journey to Recovery

"You Will Be Well!"

WHERE TO FIND THE SUPPLEMENTS IN THIS GUIDE

Vitamin C: Buffered and unbuffered from ARG/Nutricology; Buffered and Unbuffered from Ecological Formulas

B Complex (Super B): ARG /Nutricology

Hydroxy B 12: Perque Holistic Heal.com (Yasko) Amazon, Pure formulas, i-Herbs, Compound prescription for injections.

Multivitamin/Multimineral without Iron: ARG/Nutricology

Liposomal Glutathione: Lipoceutical Glutathione Life Extension.com (800) 226-2370

Glutathione Powder (For rectal use): Designs for Health

5-Methytetrahydrofolate 5-MTHF: Designs for Health, Amazon.com

Magnesium Citrate: ARG/Nutricology

Solution of Magnesium: ARG/Nutricology

Tudca: Nutricost.com or Amazon.com

Candida-Pro: Camformula.com; Natural Partners, Amazon.com, Foresthealth.com, Pure Formulas

B.I.N.D: Revelationhealth.com, dr.princetta.com/tag/bind

Omega 3 Fish Oil DHA: ARG/Nutricology

Probiotics: Klaire Labs. Natren, Pure encapsulations, Dr. Ohiro's Probiotics, ARG/Nutricology

Molybdenum Liquid: ARG/Nutricology

Pancreatic Enzymes: Pork, beef, lamb, ARG/Nutricology

Digestive Enzymes: Theramedix, sugar/starch; fat, & protein digestion

L-Citrulline: ARG/Nutricology

Tri-salts: Ecological Formulas

Organic Coconut Oil: Health food store

Organic Olive Oil: Health food store

Licorice: ARG/Nutricology

DGL: Enzymatic Therapy, Pure Encapsulations, Vital Nutrients

Lymph drainage by Desbio: Planethealth.com, Revelationhealth.com

Kidney drainage by Desbio: Planethealth.com, Revelationhealth.com

Liver drainage by Desbio: Planethealth.com, Revelationhealth.com

Immune care Candigest Plus Capsules: Immunecare.com.uk

Vitamin D: ARG/Nutricology

Full Spectrum Vitamin K: ARG/Nutricology

Dr. Clarke's Lugol's Iodine: Dr. Clarkstore.com

Zinc Gluconate: Dr. Mercola.com, NOW brand, Amazon.com, Life Extention.com

Zinc 30: Pure Encapsulations

L-Glutamine capsules: ARG/Nutricology

L-Glutamine Powder: Klaire Labs

Psyllium Sonne's #9: Health food store/online

Bentonite Sonne's #7: Health food store/online

Mastica: ARG/Nutricology

Gastromycin: ARG/Nutricology

Selenium Selenite: ARG/Nutricology

Selenium Methionine: Klaire Labs

Activated charcoal: Health food store

Taurine: ARG/Nutricology

COQ10: ARG/Nutricology

Cherry Fruit Extract: Integrative Therapeutics

Yucca: Nature's Way

L-Carnitine: ARG/Nutricology

Royal Jelly: Ecological Formulas

Grape Seed extract (Pips): ARG/Nutricology

Niacin: ARG/Nutricology

Quercetin: ARG/Nutricology

Gaba: Luckyvitamin.com, Pure Encapsulations, Douglas Labs

MarCons Nasal Test Kit: Microbiology DX

Enema kit: www.purelifeenema.com

Organic Calendula Bioactive Salve: Bodyceuticals.com, iherb.com: Amazon.com

Dr. Bernard Jensen's dry skin brush: Vitaminshoppe.com or health food store

Castor Oil: Amazon.com

Castor Oil kit (cotton or wool): Amazon.com

Plastic sheet: Whatever you can tolerate, plastic wrap

Nitrile gloves (no latex): Walgreens, CVS, or Amazon

Genetic test for CBS++: 23 and Me, Genetic Genie.org, or holisticheal.com

Sulfite strips: Holisticheal.com, or CTL Scientific strips

Pepto-Bismol: Walgreens or CVS

Organic Coffee: www.purelifeenema.com

Ceramic or glass pot: Online or local stores

Stainless steel small mesh strainer: Online or local stores or www.purelifeenema.com

Old towel: Do you own an old towel?

Hot water bottle (rubber): Walgreens or CVS

Used Sauna: Heavenly Heat with or without infrared: Craigslist. The Toxic Times Classified, e-bay, blogs, etc.

Mini-Trampoline: Amazon.com/e-Bay

Dr. Hanna's NasoPure System kit: Walgreens

SinuPulse Elite: Amazon.com

There is a store online called N.E.E.D.S. where you will find many quality supplements and books at discounted prices. Phone # is 1(800) 634-1380.

EPILOGUE

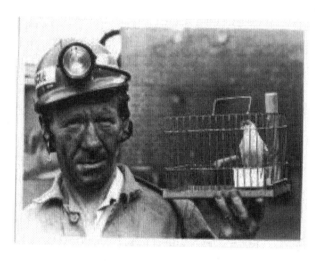

Society likens people with Chronic Illnesses as the "Canaries in the Coal Mine." The term has been used widely to describe someone or something whose sensitivity to adverse conditions makes it a useful early indicator of such conditions; something which warns of the coming of greater danger or trouble by a deterioration in their health or welfare.

Until 1986, Canaries were once regularly used in coal mining as an early warning system. Toxic gases such as carbon monoxide, methane or carbon dioxide in the mine would kill the bird before affecting the miners. Signs of distress from the bird indicated to the miners that conditions were unsafe.

Canaries were favored because their reaction to carbon monoxide was more apparent even if small quantities of the gas were present.

We, (people with chronic illnesses) are the 21st Century Canaries. There has never been more toxic air, water, and food in any century. We have been involved in a human experiment without our consent. The resulting deterioration in our health and welfare is a cautionary tale of what will happen to all beings on Earth should conditions fail to improve.

The dead Canary on the cover of my book represent people who have suffered the consequences of chemical injury and have taken their own lives. I personally knew them. I miss them. I mourn them. I dedicate this poem to them.

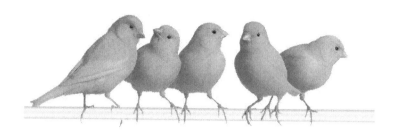

The Canary
A Poem by Rita Ferraro

We are strong, we are bold,
We are the young, we are old
Let's join our hands and chant this poem
To change the fate of humanity

We come from near, we come from far
But most of all, we're everywhere
Well send our bird into the mines
For we are one, no longer blind

We see the light, come from the dawn
Proud Sisters and Brothers, our spirits borne
We pray for you, we pray for me
Our voices be heard through eternity

The yellow bird will change their minds
We use her proudly through ups and downs
She signifies a call for arms
Our glory be heard till the end of time

REFERENCES

Rea, William J. Chemical Sensitivity. Vol.1; New York: CR Press, 1992

Rea, William J. Chemical Sensitivity. Vol.4; New York: CR Press, 1992

Caress, SM, Steinemann, AC. "Prevalence of fragrance sensitivity in the American population." Journal of Environmental Health. Mar. 2008: 46-50

Rogers, Sherry A. Detoxify or Die. New York: Prestige, 1994

Rogers, Sherry A. WELLNESS AGAINST ALL ODDS. New York: Prestige, 1994

Balch, Phyllis A. Prescription for NUTRITIONAL HEALING. New York: Penguin, 2010

Gerson, Charlotte, and Morton Walker. THE GERSON THERAPY: The Proven Nutritional Program for Cancer and Other Illnesses. New York: Kensington, 2001

Smith Lee. Coffee: Friend or Foe?: Coffee Enemas and Detoxification. Word of Nutrition and Naturopathy, 2011

Magil, MK. "Multiple Chemical Sensitivity Syndrome" American Family Physician Sept. 1998: 721-728

Kail, Conrad, Bobbi Lawrence, and Burton Goldberg. <u>ALLERGY FREE.</u> California: AlternativeMedicine.com, Inc., 2000

Yasko, Amy, and Garry Gorden. <u>The Puzzle of Autism: Putting It All Together.</u> Arizona: Matrix Development, 2004

Yasko, Amy. <u>Genetic Bypass.</u> Arizona: Matrix Development, 2005

D'Adamo, Peter J. and Catherine Whitney. <u>EAT RIGHT FOR YOUR TYPE.</u> New York: Berkley, 2016

McGarey, William A. <u>The Oil That Heals: A Physician's Successes With Castor Oil Treatments.</u> Virginia: A.R.E. Press, 1993

Davidson, Jay. <u>5 STEPS TO RESTORING HEALTH PROTOCOL.</u> Wisconsin: Jay Davidson, 2015

Gibson, Pamela. <u>Understanding and Accommodating People with MCS.</u> James Madison University. 2009

<u>Homesick: Living with Multiple Chemical Sensitivities.</u> Dir. Susan Abod. Dual Power Productions, 2013

Jensen, Bernard. <u>The Chemistry of Man.</u> Indiana: Whitman, 2012

Loomis, Howard F. Jr. <u>ENZYMES The Key to Health.</u> Vol.1. Wisconsin: 21ST CenturyNutrition, 2012

Rochlitz, Steven. Allergies and Candida. Arizona: Human Ecology Balancing Science, 2001

Thiel, Robert J. Combing Old and New: NATUROPATHY FOR THE 21ST CENTURY. Indiana: Whitman, 2000

Swi, Steve. "What is Tudca?" Evolutionary.org, 2017

Cutler, Hall Andrew. Amalgam Ilness Diagnosis and Treatment. Washington: Andrew Hall Cutler, 1999

Duncan, David. "How to Tell If You're Poisoning Yourself with Fish." Discover Magazine 19 march 2009

Hammond, David. Mercury Poisoning. Internet: CreateSpace Independent Publishing Platform, 2014

Shadowitz, Albert. The Electromagnetic Field. New York: Dover, 1988

Mercola, Joseph. "How Cellphones Cause Brain Tumors and Trigger Chronic Disease." You Tube, May 23, 2017

Mercola, Joseph. "EMF Controversy Exposed." www.merola.com: 20 Jan. 2016

Randolph, Theron and Ralph W. Moss. AN ALTERNATIVE APPROACH TO ALLERGIES THE NEW FIELD OF CLINICAL ECOLOGY. New York: Harper and Row, 1989

Scott, John. "Microwave technology: a twenty first century Trojan horse. Internet, Food Matter, 2010

"Letting a baby play on an iPad might lead to speech delays, study says" by Kelly Wallace. CNN NEWS. Atlanta, GA 2017

"Urine sulfate strips-Yasko vs. Ctl.Scientific" internet: Phoenix Rising Forum, Jan. 19, 2013

"The Concept of the Total Load" WHAT DOCTORS DON'T TELL YOU. April 1999, Vol.10, Issue 1

Haas, Elson M. "Nutritional Programs: Nutritional Programs for Allergies" internet, healthy.net, 2017

Nambudripad, Devi. "Nambudripad's Allergy Elimination Technique's" internet www.naet.com, 2017

Cutler, Ellen W. Live Free from ASTHMA and ALLERGIES: Use the BioSet System to DETOXIFY and DESENSITIZE Your Body. California: Ten Speed Press, 2007

Klinghardt, Dietrich. "Nasal Staph" BetterhealthGuy.com. "A Look Beyond Lyme." 27 April, 2013

Notes/Journal

Notes/Journal

Notes/Journal

Made in the USA
Middletown, DE
20 November 2022